The Diet Illusion

◆

THE DIET ILLUSION

A Blindingly Obvious Guide to Eating

Gaby Franklin

Illustrations by James Sillavan

Published by Lulu 2009

7 8 2 1 1 2 1

A CIP catalogue record for this book is available from the British Library.

ISBN 978 1 4452 1684 3

In memory of Fay

The Diet Illusion
A Blindingly Obvious Guide to Eating

Introduction

Introduction

This is not just another diet book. Diets, I believe, are often an illusion. This is about how really to lose weight and stay slim and healthy without giving up anything you love to eat.

How is this possible? Very simple: eat less.

You do not have to count calories. That is boring, complicated and unsustainable.

I am not a dietician and I do not believe in diets that are limiting. I am just stating the obvious – the blindingly obvious – but, strangely enough, most people do not do the obvious.

This book is for those who have truly decided that they want to lose weight and stay slim.

Really wanting to do this is the key to everything. Once you have come to this decision do not scare yourself by contemplating the size, however large or small, of the task ahead of you. Just take it meal by meal and day by day. Do not think "it will take me x years or months to lose this weight." That is too awesome. Focus on the present. As we all know staying slim is very hard, and the reasons for overeating are extremely complex. I am not attempting to analyse why people overeat. I am simply trying to help those who really want to lose weight or maintain their weight.

The aim of this book is to give you an idea of how to monitor what you eat. The suggestions are only suggestions and you can change them or adapt them to suit your lifestyle. I hope they will help you to think in a different way about losing weight and keeping it lost. It is all about taking control of your body and what goes into it. It doesn't matter if you eat loads one day; you haven't broken some rigid diet. Just eat less the next day. After a while you will know what your body needs to lose weight and to stay that way. Some of the suggestions may seem impossible for you to do. If so, ignore them, but remember they are only there to help you eat less of what you like – if only a little less of it!

Each of the first ten chapters has a few key rules. They are followed by a list of tips that should help you implement them. Once you are happy with how you feel the book goes on to help you retain a healthy body. There are some answers to some obvious questions that often remain unasked. And along the way we follow the story of a Hassled, Overweight, Peckish Eater – HOPE – someone you might just recognise.

I have spent my adult life following the rules in this book and they have worked. These rules have evolved over many years as I watched my overweight mother try numerous diets. She lost weight and put it back on many times. I promised myself I would never get to her size but I would eat and enjoy each meal.

She never controlled her weight properly and died too young of a heart attack. This book is in her memory.

1

SHOPPING

What you buy is what you eat.

Hope is a schoolteacher with two children. Her daughter is a typical teenager and her son, the much wanted afterthought, is three. Each January she always means to lose about 14 pounds (6 kilos) by the time she goes on her summer holiday. Her life is very full, as you can imagine. She typically collects her son from the childminder after work and hurries to the local supermarket. All she really wants to do is go home and have a cup of tea; instead she finds herself with her son either in the trolley or tugging at her hand as she heads for the aisles. Although she has a shopping list the trolley soon fills up with quick-to-cook ready meals and sugar- and salt-laden snacks that her out-of-control son sneaks into the trolley when her back is turned. Her son is complaining, playing up and hungry, so she ends up giving him one of the chocolate bars she had not even meant to buy!

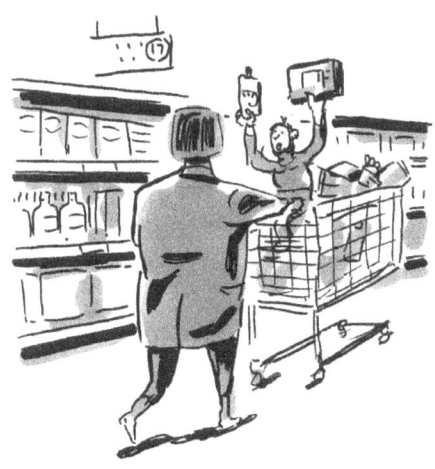

Hope is not doing anything that might seem terribly wrong, but her whole shopping experience could be improved with a few changes and a different attitude. So, if anything Hope does sounds familiar, or not – read on.

You might not have thought of shopping as an integral part of losing weight, but it is. Food shops are full of choices and you need to make sure that the purchases you make will help you to achieve your goal of either losing weight or maintaining the weight you have lost.

Here are a few simple rules, followed by some tips on how to help you to stick to them. Obviously, the more weight you have to lose the stricter you can be. But remember: it is better to lose weight slowly and change the way you eat for good.

What you buy is what you eat.

This is the most important thing to remember when you are food shopping. If you do not buy it you will not be able to eat it!

This may seem obvious – and it is – but it is crucial in helping you start your new eating pattern. By thinking of what you will buy you are focusing on what you will be eating, and getting yourself into the right frame of mind for all that follows.

If you do a weekly shop do not buy more than you plan to eat. If you shop daily the same principle applies.

I know many people like to buy in bulk. This is fine for cleaning products, but if you want to eat less it really helps to buy only what you plan to use. If there is an abundance of food at home obviously the temptation to eat it is greater – so make it easier for yourself and buy only what you need. You may think that buying the larger size of something is more economical. Wrong. You end up spending more and eating more!

Factor in time for shopping. If you hurry you are more likely to do a bad shop.

This again sounds obvious, but in practice it is often ignored. It may be hard to give yourself longer to shop, but it is worth trying very hard to do so. The less time you have the more likely you are to pick things up without really thinking whether or not they are what you really want to eat.

If you do not have much time for shopping it helps to make a list. This stops you wandering around aimlessly. It is also good to try to shop in a supermarket that you know. You will avoid wasting time looking for things and give you time to focus on buying what you want.

Try not to shop with children if possible.

I love my children but they do try to sneak the most unhealthy, calorie-laden items into the basket. Not taking yours might be hard and could mean changing when you shop. The change will be worth it. You might even begin to enjoy food shopping, if you have always found it a chore. Look at it as time for you – when you can decide what you want to eat. Treat yourself to something small: bath stuff, flowers or anything that makes you feel pampered.

If you do have to take children, make sure that they have a healthy snack to eat while they are sitting in the trolley, or some small toy to occupy them if they are going to be mobile while you shop. Once they are older you could enlist their help in finding healthy things to eat that you would all like. This is a chance to educate them into eating well.

Only shop online if you have to.

Unless you really detest food shopping or have no time I would not recommend that you shop online as you lose a certain amount of control over exactly what is delivered – the substitutes are not always great. Besides, you get good exercise walking around a supermarket.

Shopping tips

These tips work for me and maybe some of them will work for you. You might buy completely different things on your shop. The knack is to buy a lot of what you like that is good for you and a little of what you like that you know is not exactly great. Just remind yourself there are no good and bad foods, just foods you should eat more or less of. It has probably been drummed into you for years that there are definitely good and bad foods. It is hard to live your life like that. Sometimes we all need a little of what we fancy! Most of these tips you probably already know but you might not always apply them when shopping.

A little of anything will not make you fat!

◆ If you are a snacker then buy healthy snacks: fruit or vegetables that can be eaten raw, little packets of raisins or such-like. If you need to have snacks such as crisps then get low-fat ones and only a very small amount. If you are trying to lose weight and have no kids in your household try not to buy crisps but stock up on carrots, mushrooms or cauliflower or any vegetable that is good raw.

♦ If you enjoy chicken, buy skinned breasts. The white meat is slightly better for you. If you prefer dark meat then it is better not to eat the skin. But obviously if you love crispy skin have a very little bit!

♦ Red meat should be bought with as little fat as possible. Always cut off excess fat before cooking. Escalopes of most meats are a good option as they are usually lean and come in small pieces.

♦ Buy as few ready meals as possible. Unless you are really pushed for time I would not recommend them. They are expensive, generally full of salt and preservatives, often quite high in calories and not particularly good for you. Obviously if you are really in a rush and you have a craving for one – buy it! Just check what is in it.

♦ Go easy on salami (there is a lot of fat in most types – you can see it). Thin, lean ham is good.

♦ Buy berries, fruit or yogurts for desserts. If you like fruit this is always the best dessert option. Go easy on bananas, grapes and cherries.

♦ If you must have fizzy drinks limit what you buy and get used to all the diet versions. I do not like to push buying the diet version of things, but when it comes to Coke and other fizzy drinks I change my tune!

♦ Buy as much salad and vegetables as you think you can eat – only if you like all this greenery, though.

♦ Obviously buy semi-skimmed or skimmed milk.

♦ Do not always buy the very low-fat item: if you like cottage cheese then go for the regular kind if you prefer it, not the very low-fat sort. The idea is that you enjoy your food.

♦ Try to buy one different food item, preferably a healthy one, each week. This just adds a bit of variety.

♦ If you have the time, plan in advance what you want for meals. This might only take ten minutes but it will be well worth it and save you time in the long run.

♦ When buying fruit, buy small sizes of apples or bananas etc. Many supermarkets sell lunch-box sizes.

♦ Cereals can be good if they do not have too much sugar and loads of additives and colouring. Check the content carefully and if you have children try to introduce them to plainer cereals. As a rule fluorescent colours are not the most healthy.

♦ If you must have chocolates or biscuits then buy one packet only. Rich tea biscuits seem to have the least of everything bad! Only buy them if you are sure you can stop at one biscuit or one square of chocolate. Be honest with yourself.

♦ If you have a love of good cheese, do not cut it out but severely limit what you buy. Mini sizes of cheese are good.

♦ Opt for the smallest package of most things,

especially if you live alone and there is no one to finish up the leftovers other than you.

◆ Go easy on dips, as they are often heavier than you think.

◆ Any sort of fresh fish is good. An alternative to battered fish is breaded – slightly better for you. Avoid buying tinned fish (like tuna) in oil. Tuna in brine is better.

◆ If you can, opt for tomato-based pasta sauces not cream ones.

◆ Buy food as close to its natural produced state as possible.

After rethinking how she did her shopping Hope had a better experience…

She decided to change her shopping time to one that would suit her. She bribed her teenage daughter into looking after her little brother. She sat down with a cup of tea before she left. And she wrote her shopping list. She arrived at the supermarket feeling surprisingly relaxed and ready to glide peacefully round the aisles. She bought all the essentials, then spent time in the bath section choosing a lavender soak. That was followed by treating herself to the latest John Grisham novel. The bill was a surprise, less than normal. Why? More on her and less on expensive junk foods. She arrived home happy. Well much happier than her daughter, who was stressed out and ratty after looking after her darling little brother!

2
BREAKFAST

Breakfast is the most important meal of the day.

Rush! That word summed up Hope's mornings. She just about managed to get herself and her family up on time. Everyone was yelling at each other about something and breakfast seemed always eaten on the go – if at all. She usually picked something up just before going into work. The rest of the family sometimes managed to grab something, like a bowl of cereal, and eat it standing up by the counter. The weekends were only slightly better as everyone slept in and then rushed to get off to their particular activity. She could not remember the last time she sat down for a leisurely breakfast. Maybe in her dreams!

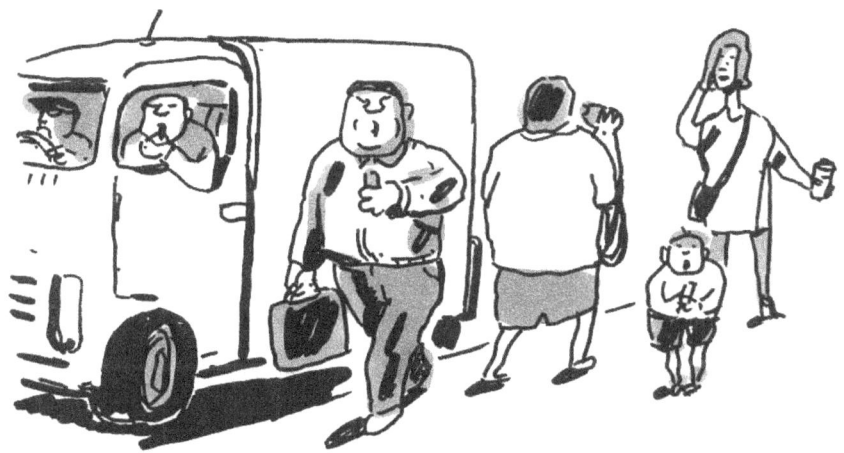

Does anything about Hope's morning sound a tiny bit like yours? If so, your start to the day is not good, especially if you want to lose weight or maintain your hard-won figure. Breakfast is a meal to be eaten and enjoyed.

To enjoy breakfast you might have to make a change or two to your routine but it will be worth it. I so often hear people say proudly that they have had nothing to eat all day. You will not lose weight or keep weight off in this way. All that happens is that you are ravenous at the end of the day and eat too much too quickly. If you eat too little your body will use less energy so that the moment you begin eating normally again you will put on weight. That is the diet-binge regimen that this book is trying to help you break, and having breakfast is integral to everything. Trust me: if you have not eaten since supper you will be hungry and want to get up to have breakfast!

This is the most important meal of the day.

Making this an important meal might seem really difficult for many people. For some this will involve big changes. But how you start your day is crucial, especially if you are thinking about your weight. You have the morning to digest and work off your breakfast. If you are radically cutting down to lose a lot of weight it might seem appealing and give fast results to miss breakfast altogether and still manage to undereat during the rest of the day; so be it, if it is helpful to you. But remember that when you achieve your goal you should start to have breakfast, as it really does set you up for the day. So maybe you could manage from day one to have something even if you do not want to – it will be better for sustaining your weight loss.

Give yourself enough time to eat breakfast.

This might mean getting up a little earlier if you can. It will also mean that you might have to become a little more organised – I know that can be hard but it helps give you more time. Preparing things for breakfast the previous night is helpful, especially on weekdays. I am not suggesting that you come down to cold soggy toast. Maybe get out the plates and cutlery that you need. This might seem a bit pedantic but however many minutes you can save in the morning will make a difference. At the weekends you will probably have more time so really plan a long, leisurely meal. You can plan it by making sure you have good things to eat, good things to read (if you are alone) and good company.

Do not to leave home or start work feeling hungry.

If you leave your home feeling hungry you will have food on your mind – this is not good. So no hunger pangs when you walk out of the front door.

Sit down to eat.

This might seem obvious but so many people just grab something on the go. A better way is to sit down and savour the meal. You are more likely to remember you have eaten and not want to eat again so soon.

Breakfast tips

♦ Pour yourself a big glass of water and make sure you drink it. Water is just so good for everything. You can never have enough.

♦ If you like to eat cereal then choose one that does not have too much added sugar (as mentioned in "shopping"). Really study the packet. If it says it is low in cholesterol this does not mean it is particularly good for you, as most cereal does not need to have fats/cholesterol. Try to steer your kids to healthier cereals. Remember to limit your-self to a small portion – a handful is a good amount!

♦ Never have full-fat milk with your cereal. Nobody needs it except babies

♦ If you like butter on your toast, have a little. If you like to have lashings of the stuff then maybe look at finding a low-fat, low-calorie spread that does not taste horrible. Best of all learn to spread thinly.

♦ Cut bread thinly or buy a thin-cut loaf.

- If you like to spread your jam thinly then stick with the real thing. But if you like mountains of the stuff then look for a low-calorie one that you can stomach and try to cut down the layers! The best thing is to eat less jam if you can.

- If you have juice to start your day then make sure there is no added sugar or any-thing else nasty in it. When you have a lot of time squeeze yourself an orange or grapefruit juice – much healthier and much tastier. A great weekend treat.

- If you are an egg person then try to opt for a boiled or poached one – they are both better than fried. Obviously the odd fried egg is not bad especially if you just want to maintain your weight.

- Fried food is really best avoided but if you have a craving for sausages and bacon on a weekend morning then use very little oil, and once you have fried them place each one on a piece of kitchen roll just before eating – this will absorb some of the fat. Only ever have one sausage and one rasher of bacon.

♦ Eat slowly. Try to get a family member to eat with you – if possible – or else study the paper! Being occupied when you are eating helps to slow the process and that is good.

♦ If you take sugar in your tea and coffee, try not to. If that is impossible then try to cut down or have a low calorie-sweetener.

♦ If you have the time and energy, vary what you have. My favourite breakfast is avocado on toast with a tad of butter and some lemon squeezed over it. This is not a low-calorie item but I love it and avocado con-tains loads of good stuff. Find your ultimate breakfast!

♦ If you like to start your day with a croissant, go for the low-fat variety. If it is a big one – split it with someone or cut it in half and make it last two days. Put it in the oven or toaster on second usage.

♦ Treat a *pain au chocolat* the same way as a croissant, but be even meaner with yourself.

♦ Muffins can be bought in mini sizes – these are the ones you should go for.

♦ Fruit is a good way to start the day.

These are just a few pointers to get you started. Most of them are fairly obvious but there might be a few that help a bit.

There is nothing complicated about any of it. Just eat LESS.

Hope decided there were going to be some changes to early-morning life…

The alarm clock went off half an hour earlier. She leapt out of bed, curious about her new breakfast plans. She had a very peaceful, unrushed shower. Once she was ready to face the day she woke up the rest of the family, telling them breakfast would be ready in fifteen minutes. She had worried that she might not get the support she needed for her eating changes. But everyone complied with the change and actually enjoyed it. She had always thought that she had a supportive family. Now she knew she did. There was time for toast, tea and conversation before everyone dashed out. As Hope travelled to work she could feel herself smiling. What a civilised start to the day!

3
LUNCH

Never miss lunch.

By lunchtime the old Hope was completely ravenous as breakfast had been virtually non-existent. As usual there was a pile of work still waiting to be done. Lunch would have to be at her desk with sandwiches. No time even to go out to get them. Her assistant brought her in a huge baguette filled with chicken, salad and lashings of butter and salad cream and some crisps and a chocolate bar to keep her going through the afternoon. She devoured the sandwich within minutes and then worked her way, straight after, through the crisps and chocolate. By three o'clock she couldn't even remember if she had had any lunch!

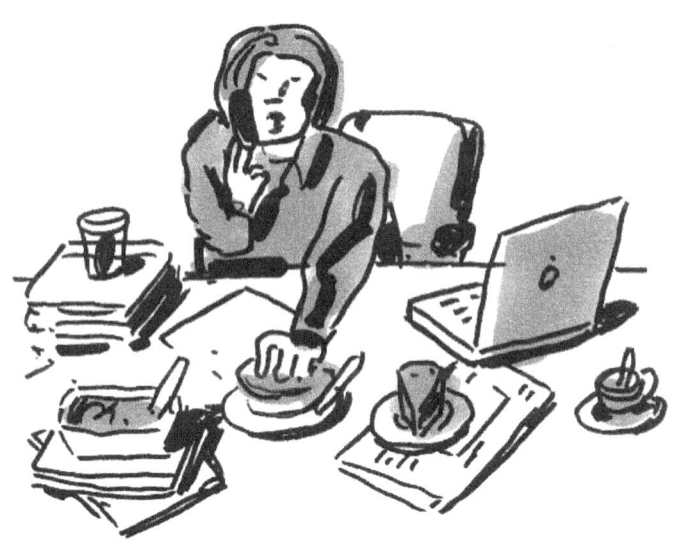

Hope did not miss lunch but she did not get it right! Hope – the old Hope that is – would think about lunch because she was starving after having had virtually no breakfast. With just a little thought she could have avoided her mistakes.

Lunch can be a hard meal to do properly. There are so many different kinds: work lunches, sandwich/snack lunches, lunch on your own, lunch with friends, weekend lunches, quick lunches, leisurely lunches.

This is a meal that you should take the time to think about. You have to think what meals are either side of it to decide how much you should have. To give you an example, I work from home and am a creature of habit when it comes to food. Most weekdays I have plain pasta with freshly cut up tomatoes, salt, pepper, olive oil and a little Parmesan. If I know I am going to have a big supper then I simply make less pasta & have slightly more tomatoes. Very simple. As I keep saying: just eat less.

Never miss lunch.

If you have no lunch you are probably going to eat more at suppertime. As with breakfast, there is a tendency (especially if you are trying to shed weight quickly) to feel good if you miss lunch. This is a mistake. Try to have something, however little. It might appear to slow down rapid weight loss a tiny bit but for the future having the right lunch is a good habit to get into.

If you are going to have a big three-course meal, this is the one to have it at.

This does not mean that lunch should always be three courses! It means that it is better to have your big meal at lunchtime. Of course, this might not always be possible. But when it is, do it. It means you will have longer to digest it and burn it off. But if your life does not make the time for this, do not worry, just carry on eating less at all meals.

Make sure you are really aware you have had lunch.

This might seem a crazy notion, that you are not aware you have had lunch – but it is very common. People will often say "oh I had no lunch today except a bit of sandwich and some crisps". This IS lunch, of course, but because of the way, or when, they might have eaten it they discount it as a meal. It is easy to be aware of having had lunch if it is at a restaurant or with friends but if you eat on your own it really helps to make it separate from what you are doing. For example, if you are at home make sure you sit down, use a plate, knife, fork and glass. Do not open the fridge door, grab something, stand up and eat something quickly with your hands. If that is you, then try to change!

Lunch tips

♦ If you are stuck in the office at your desk with your lunch then clear some space on your desk, stop working and either talk to a work mate while you are eating or find a book or magazine to read. This makes lunch feel like a proper meal.

♦ If you are having a sandwich lunch make sure you give yourself time to enjoy it. It might only be a sandwich, but it is still your midday meal.

♦ If you work near a park or open space and often have sandwich lunches, try to eat them in the park either with a work mate, personal music system or a good book. That way you will still be occupied when you finish eating. And in peaceful surroundings (this is obviously a good-weather option).

♦ If you are having sandwiches it is better either to make them at home or to get them freshly made in a cafe. Prepackaged ones are the worst as you have less control over what is in them. Try not to have to have butter on the bread if a cafe is making them, they always seem to put lashings on! I often order a tuna or chicken salad sandwich but always try to have less chicken or meat and more salad and little mayonnaise. You might prefer cheese, in which case you should ask for it to be cut thinly.

◆ Lunch at friends can be hard if you are trying to lose weight. But you still want to enjoy yourself, so just try everything you fancy but no seconds! If there is something that looks really heavy just eat a little and if vegetables are on offer and you like them fill your plate up with these. Make sure the vegetables are not laced with loads of butter before you pile them on, though.

◆ Business lunches are often at restaurants (see restaurant section). At least you have the choice here.

◆ If you have a big lunch at the weekend always try to go for a walk afterwards.

◆ Try not to have lunch too late. Too late means you are ravenous and therefore likely to eat too much too fast. Bad.

- Soup is a good alternative to sandwich lunches at work. They are becoming easier and easier to get. Stay away from the very creamy kind and check the content if you want to lose weight.

- Salads are a good lunch food but make sure that the dressing is not laced with loads of calories and always get it on the side. Stay clear of pasta salad, potato salad – in fact any creamy salad. If the creamy ones are what you like then do not think of them as salads, but as pasta or potato dishes served cold with a sauce, and eat accordingly. Oil, vinegar, salt and pepper is always the best option for a salad dressing – if you like it!

- Sushi boxes are readily available in most supermarkets. These are healthy and good. Just check the calorie content of the pack.

- If you are at work try to buy your lunch for yourself. That way you have total control over what you get.

- Try not to have too much alcohol at lunch, except at the weekends, if you must. Alcohol is full of calories – be aware of this. If you want to lose weight try to cut it down to the minimum that you are happy with.

◆ If you are out shopping, walking, cycling or doing any strenuous exercise remember to stop and eat lunch.

◆ The important thing is to like what you have, not to have it just because it seems healthy. Enjoy – even if it is less!

Hope decided more changes were on the cards. The next change was lunch…

She had been really active before leaving for work and made herself a packed lunch of a tuna and cucumber sandwich on brown bread with a smidgeon of mayonnaise instead of butter. For dessert she had included a satsuma and a square of her favourite dark orange organic chocolate. She made a point of clearing her desk around lunchtime, getting out her goodies and reading the paper. Having finished, she nipped out to the local coffee bar to get a skimmed milk cappuccino. Suddenly, as if on command, the sun came out. She spent the rest of her lunchtime lying in the park having her coffee and watching the ducks. She was ready for whatever the afternoon had to throw at her.

4
SUPPER

The lighter the better.

Hope, of the old eating habits, arrived home starving after her day of not eating too well. Everyone was there when she arrived. They were starving as well. She had planned to make a healthy supper of baked fish and vegetables. No one, including her, wanted to wait while the fish was cleaned and the vegetables prepared. So, guess what, into the microwave went an array of ready meals. Creamy mushroom risotto to start, with beef in a cream and wine sauce with mashed cheddar cheese potatoes to follow. And it was all washed down with some chilled beer. She had even managed to devour a packet of tortilla chips, with a tub of sour cream dip before the ready meals made it to the table. She offered everyone fruit for dessert but they had already spotted the praline and toffee ice cream in the freezer. The fruit never left the bowl and the tub of ice cream never made it back to the freezer. The ice cream was just too tempting for Hope and her hungry family.

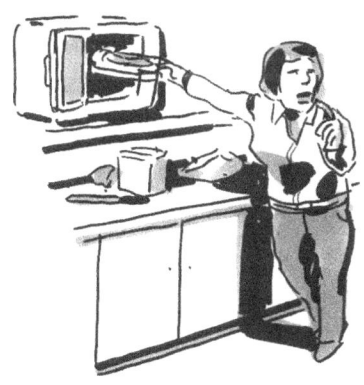

Hope went to bed feeling full and I am sure she did not sleep well. She ate too much of the wrong things at the wrong time!

You obviously should have supper but if you really want to lose weight you should cut it down. Even if you are at your target weight it is never good to eat a very heavy meal at the end of the day. It often just lies on your stomach and you end up not having a very sound night's sleep. It is best to go bed not feeling bloated. If you feel bloated you have eaten too much.

The lighter the better.

This is hard as supper is the most sociable meal and often the one you have the most time for. But if you really want to lose some weight it is important to eat a light supper. That might sound difficult but it does not need to be, especially if you have been eating correctly all day.

Try to have supper as early as possible.

The reasons for doing this are obvious – the earlier you eat the more time you have to work off the meal and the less likely you are to go to bed feeling bloated. Plus the earlier you eat the less likely you are to need a teatime snack to tide you over until supper. If you can't change your eating time then at least make sure that you really eat less and try to walk about a bit after eating.

The less you make the less you eat.

Try not to make a lot of food. As you know by now it is not good for anyone to eat a lot before they go to bed.

Try to make supper the last food before breakfast.

After supper really is the worst time to snack. If you can be disciplined and not snack after you have eaten you will really feel the benefits. I know that watching TV in the evening can make you feel like tea with something. Have the tea but try to skip the something. This can be hard but give it a try!

Supper tips

♦ Try to eat supper as slowly as you can, as you should have the time. If you are a fast eater try taking a mouthful, putting your cutlery down and waiting a few seconds before taking another bite.

♦ If you know you are going to eat late – have a healthy snack early on in the evening so you are not completely starving by the time you sit down. By having a small snack you are less likely to overeat over late!

♦ After eating, have a walk. It need not be a long walk, just around the block. Eating and then going straight to bed is not a good idea: you can end up sleeping badly and feeling very bloated.

♦ Once you have eaten and intend to eat no more, brush your teeth. That is a good way of saying to yourself that there is no more food until breakfast.

♦ Go very easy on desserts. A couple of bites are more than enough.

◆ Fruit is always the best end to a meal.

◆ Keep your alcohol to a minimum and drink plenty of water instead.

◆ If you have kids and have to feed them earlier, try not to pick at their leftovers (leftovers are a big no-no!) Get their plates cleared away very quickly. If you have to sit with them, make yourself a drink of water/tea/coffee and resist trying their food.

◆ If you are cooking for a dinner party, be aware of any tasting that goes on before you sit down to eat. If you have already tried most of the dishes, serve yourself a very meagre portion. Be honest with yourself.

◆ If you are having people for dinner or are out to dinner, be aware of any snacks you have with drinks – have some if you must, but a tiny amount and try to keep away from peanuts.

◆ If eating more than one course, make sure you have time to digest the starter before the main course. By giving yourself time to digest each course you should feel less bloated at the end of the meal. This digesting time is particularly important at night.

♦ Do not have seconds. This might sound a bit strict but it is particularly important especially if you want to lose weight. If you are a person who usually has seconds then by cutting them out you should really feel the difference.

♦ Leave the food area as soon as supper is cleared up. If you are out of reach of food you are less likely to be tempted.

♦ Try to do something after supper other than watch TV – take a long luxurious bath, read, play a game, go for a walk or whatever else you enjoy.

♦ Try to eat the most healthy, least heavy food that you can for this meal.

♦ Try to give up having supper in front of the TV.

♦ Enjoy the feeling of not having a full stomach at the end of the meal.

- ♦ Just another reminder. This really is the meal where you should eat much, much less.

- ♦ Enjoy your supper!

Hope was ready to make changes to how she ate at suppertime…

Hope arrived home from the childminder with her toddler, who thankfully was very tired and fell asleep straight after his bath. Hope had an hour before she was due to go out and she planned to make the most of it. She had a cup of tea and a plain biscuit and then headed to the bathroom. After luxuriating in a lavender bath she was ready for an evening out. She was meeting her husband and some good friends at the local bistro. She arrived feeling relaxed and ready for a leisurely meal. Her tea and biscuit (one biscuit!) had taken the edge off her appetite. She ordered Parma ham followed by giant grilled shrimps with a green salad. She persuaded her husband to share a mango sorbet with her for dessert. Since she was driving home, she stuck to water and a few sips of white wine. The meal lasted ages as there was a lot of gossiping going on. She really did not feel at all bloated and slept like a log.

5

SNACKS

Think before you snack.

Hope had been cleaning up in the kitchen and had a rare few minutes to herself. She was about to go to watch the news on TV when she noticed a half-eaten box of chocolates on the table. She could not resist one, and then another, and before she knew it the box was virtually empty! After the chocolates she felt thirsty so had the remainder of a can of Fanta that her daughter had brought in after school. As there were only a couple of chocolates left in the box she thought she might as well take them into the TV room and finish the box while watching the news.

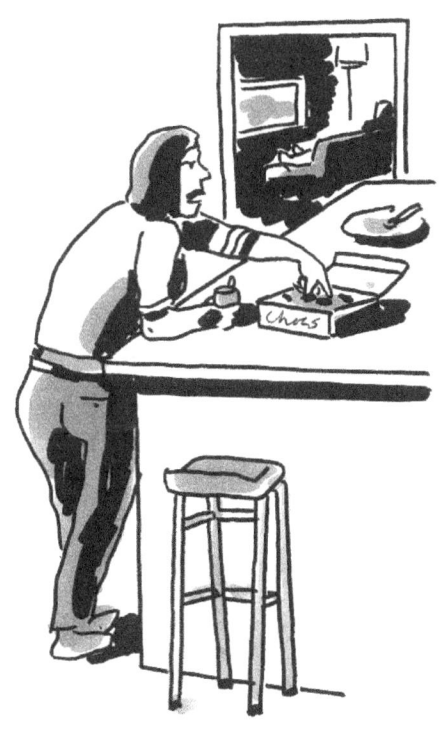

Everything Hope did was wrong. She had not even been hungry but ate just because the box of chocolates was there. Even if she had been peckish, chocolate was not the thing to have, especially in such quantity. When her thirst kicked in she took the nearest thing to hand, which was also not good.

As you can see snacks are a real danger area. Hope's example shows how easy it is to make mistakes. I am not saying never snack. I am just saying snack on the right things for the right reasons.

Think before you snack.

Ask yourself the question: "Am I really hungry or am I just in the kitchen/food shop and fancy popping something in my mouth?" Most times you will answer that you are not hungry but are thinking of eating for no particular reason other than boredom, comfort or even just because food is right in front of you and you cannot resist the temptation. If you really are hungry then snack, but in the right way!

Remember your snacks.

This may sound obvious, but most people tend to forget their snacks as quickly as they have eaten them. Often this is because you have a snack so quickly that it does not register as a significant piece of food, although it usually is. Being aware that you have snacked will remind you to eat less at your next meal.

Stay away from temptation.

This can be hard to do but well worth attempting. Try not to hang around the kitchen unless you have to. Keep snacks out of the area where you are working, watching TV or reading. Try not to have loads of unhealthy snacks lying around the house. Do not buy them kidding yourself that they are for the other people in the house and not you. Take temptation away. Hopefully what you do not see you do not want!

Write down what you eat.

This might seem a very extreme idea. It is only a suggestion. It works for some people, especially when it comes to snacking. Writing down what you have for breakfast, lunch or supper can be simple once you get in the routine. But if you have to write down every time you snack as well it could become tedious. So this is only for those who like obsessive note taking. It might make you think even harder –

do I really want this? Keeping a small notebook with a record of what you eat can be interesting. You might notice that certain things have different effects on how you are feeling. Or you might find the entire notion of keeping a notebook freakish – if so, don't!

Snack tips

♦ The best snacks are apples, pears, citrus fruits and raw cut-up vegetables. If cut-up vegetables alone do not appeal then try them with a tiny weeny bit of dip, mayonnaise or cottage cheese. Try low-fat dips.

♦ Dried fruit is also a healthy snack in moderation – maybe as little as three or four pieces of apricots or one of those lunch-size raisin packets.

♦ If you crave a salty snack, try cutting up a tomato and sprinkling salt over it. If tomatoes do not satisfy your craving and you still want crisps or something along those lines, look for a small low-fat pack and eat only about one-third or less of the contents.

♦ Sandwiches should not really be thought of as a snack, as they are more a light meal, especially the prepackaged ones. You think that a sandwich sounds healthy but it really depends what it has in it. If you just take a look at the calorie content of most supermarket sandwiches you will be amazed. I am not saying: no sandwiches. I am just reminding you that if you really want one, be aware that it is a "big" piece of food. If you crave bread as part of a snack then cut a very thin slice and have it with a light spread or nothing. If the only bread item available to you is a pre-made sandwich, then only eat a quarter or half of it – max; a couple of bites would be even better!

♦ Drinks are also snacks, so go easy on endless cups of tea and coffee with milk. Black coffee or tea is better, and water is even better.

♦ Go very easy on pre-dinner snacks with drinks. Try to steer clear of the nuts and crisps but feel free to overdose on veggies or olives. Remember what quantity of snacks you have eaten when you are having the meal.

♦ A real danger time for oversnacking is when you watch TV. Try not to have stuff to eat at hand so that if you do snack at least you have to get up and get it! Try not to snack in front of the TV: you are less likely to be aware of how much you have eaten.

♦ At the cinema, if you must have popcorn then get the smallest size and share it with everyone. Anyone who complains about sharing – get a spare cup and give them their own bit. No one needs to stuff themselves with popcorn or sweets.

♦ If you are around when your kids come in from school and they have snacks that you are often unable to resist, then I suggest that you leave the room or decide you are going to have a tiny portion of what they are having. As soon as you have finished, leave the room and do not return until they are finished. If you are worried about your children overeating the wrong things, prepare their snacks in advance- that way you can monitor slightly better what they eat.

♦ Try to reward toddlers with healthy stuff instead of all the usual sweets and crisps: that way they will hopefully not get you to bring temptation into the home. They could be so happy with a plate of carrots – if you are really lucky!

♦ If you are trying to lose a lot of weight then see if you can cut out snacks or only have really, really healthy ones. If you do snack too much, simply have less to eat at other times of the day.

♦ If you are about to snack, think how long it is to the next meal and try to last out.

♦ Do not deny yourself chocolate or sweets. Just have one square, one sweet, one bite. Get to enjoy "one"!

Now Hope wanted to deal with her snacking habits…

Hope arrived home to find her daughter had just entertained half the neighbourhood. The kitchen table was littered with half-eaten crisp packets, biscuits, chocolates and cans of Coke. She quickly put the half-eaten crisps in the bin and stored the rest of it. She was feeling a bit peckish but her daughter's snacks were not on her menu. She got out her bowl of sliced carrots. She sliced an apple and mixed it up with cottage cheese, put on some music and settled down with her snacks and book. As soon as she finished she woke her son and took him to the park for some active playing. She felt a bit peckish again while she was watching television, later that night. This time she went into the kitchen and realised that she was not really hungry. Just a bit bored because she had zapped through all the channels and the best available was "Desperate Housewives" and now it was the break. Feeling really pleased with herself she went back to the desperation of the soap-opera housewives!

6

TAKE-OUTS

Do the ordering yourself.

The traffic had been terrible and everyone arrived home late feeling hungry, tired and in no mood to cook. The unreformed Hope grabbed the first available take-out menu from the notice board, which happened to be a pizza one. She quickly called and ended up ordering far too much as they had a two-for-one special with free soft drinks (the non-diet variety). By the time all the pizzas arrived everyone was completely ravenous. Hope ate far too much too quickly in front of the TV. The pizzas stayed in the TV room for the rest of the evening as nobody could be bothered to take them into the kitchen. Hope continued to nibble until everything was gone. Naturally she felt utterly bloated!

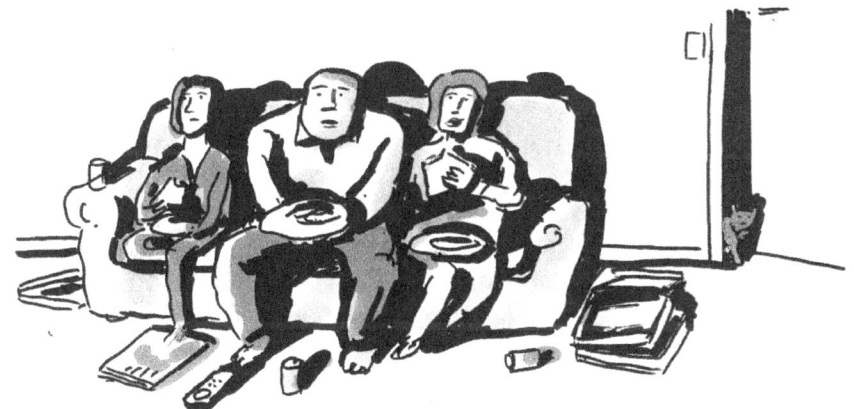

Again Hope has got it wrong – bad timing, bad food and bad amount!

Take-outs are fine once in a while but you really do have to give them some thought. I have some basic rules when ordering any take-outs and then there are some tips that can be helpful when ordering specific types of meal.

Do the ordering yourself.

Clearly if you order you have more control over the dishes and the size of them. The more you order the more you eat. You can approach the ordering as you would in a restaurant: the more unhealthy the food is, the less you should order. If you are ordering for a few people, check that they like your choices or you could end up with most of it to yourself.

Always share.

What I mean by this is that it is not advisable to or-der a take-out just for yourself as most portions are too big for one and you would end up overeating. If you decide to order for one try to go for a healthy option or something that will keep for a while in the fridge. Or be prepared ruthlessly to allocate yourself a portion and then put the rest in the bin.

Indulge in novelty not quantity.

Remember the idea is still to enjoy food! Although my mantra is "eat less" that does not mean that you should not experiment. Where you can, try something new or, better still, order a small selection. This is easily done with Japanese, Chinese or Thai food, especially if there are a few of you eating.

Take-out tips

♦ **Bagels**. Bagels in themselves are not terrible if you have a yen for carbohydrates. The problem is what is inside them. Plain cream cheese spread very thinly with smoked salmon is an OK meal. If you pick one up from a specialty bagel shop ask for it to be made up with half a portion of filling.

♦ **Chinese**. Have plain boiled rice, not fried. Try not to have battered meat. Go for steamed vegetables, not fried. Have few prawn crackers. Try not to eat much of the skin with the Peking duck in pancakes, but you can go very heavy on all the greenery that goes with it. Go easy on all sauces. Chicken and fish are lighter than beef and duck. Just enjoy the tastes but limit the quantity.

♦ **Coffee bars**. Always have skimmed or semi-skimmed milk. Lattes are higher in calories than cappuccinos, espresso is OK – as is any coffee without milk and sugar. The same applies to teas. Coffee bars often sell cakes, muffins and sandwiches. Check the content of the sandwiches and go easy on the sweet stuff. As I always say – share it!

♦ **Crepes**. These vary hugely depending what is inside them. A simple light one with little sugar and lemon is OK if you have only one or less. Crepes stuffed with cheese and cream are not advisable if you want to lose weight.

♦ **Fish and chips**. Obviously this is not the best meal if you want to lose weight but there will be times when you are faced with a bag of soggy chips and fish. Remember: the bigger the chips the less fried surface area there is. Never ever eat a whole portion of chips. If you want to lose weight you should not have more than about half a dozen. If that is impossible them cut back on something else.

Battered fish is so bad: I remove the batter and just eat a bit of the fish. If that is too rigid then have a couple of bites – maximum. The pickles in fish and chip shops are fat-free, acidic, but low in calories and something that you can eat in moderation without worrying.

- **Fried chicken**. Another really fatty meal. I always take the skin off but then the chicken underneath is not so great. You could opt for a chicken burger. The meat is still fried but not always coated in batter. Only eat a bite or two of the bun. Eat fried chicken rarely; if you have a craving, have a little and be aware of what else you have eaten that day. Do not be afraid to put half of this meal in the bin; it is better there than in your stomach!

- **Greek**. Greek salads are OK – just eat a third to half of the feta in them. Grilled chicken or prawn kebabs are healthyish. (Mezze – see restaurants)

- **Hamburgers**. These are not particularly good, as you know, so always go for the basic simplest one and then try to split it with someone – or leave half. Chips in fast-food hamburger takes-outs are often fatty as they are long and skinny. So greasier. The salads are not so healthy either as the dressing often carries more calories than the plain hamburger. Never have a supersized portion unless you are sharing ONE portion with friends, as many friends as possible.

- **Hot dogs**. A few bites will not be too terrible if you are in the cold at a football match or at the cinema. Not the best food to have though. Again, never eat a whole one unless it is your whole meal.

- **Ice cream**. If you really crave one on a hot day, go for either a frozen yogurt or sorbet. If the above do not do it for you, have only one scoop, and if you go for the very creamy rich variety – praline, pecan etc – share one scoop!

- **Indian**. Tandoori is relatively healthy. Curries and vegetable dishes in sauce are not so good as they are often too greasy – so only have a little and never mop up the remains on the dish. Rice is OK, as is a little bit of nan if you crave carbohydrates.

- **Japanese**. This is not a bad take-out food. Most of it is OK. Just do not eat too much because you think it is OK! Sushi is probably the most healthy. Raw fish is good. As you know by now, most raw stuff is OK. Obviously do not take this literally. Raw chicken is really not a delight!

- **Juice bars**. Fresh juices are full of good stuff but they can be very filling and very high in calories. Go for carrot and tomato as opposed to a creamy berry concoction. Share one if part of a meal.

- **Mexican**. This is quite heavy food, especially Tex Mex. It is laced with sour cream and guacamole. Eat very small quantities of most Mexican food.

- **Pizza**. Always go for thin crust as this has less cheese and dough and is generally less heavy. The simpler the pizza the better. Meat tends to really bulk them out. But again if you have to have pepperoni then go easy. If you want to lose weight, one to one-and-a-half slices is enough. A lot of pizza places offer celery and wings with dips; steer clear of these. You think they sound healthy but the dips are high in calories as is the sauce that the wings are covered in.

- **Sandwich bars**. Just go for light fillings – tuna, prawn, salad, and Parma ham. Ask for little butter or mayonnaise.

♦ **Thai**. This is not too heavy – just stay away from the deep-fried stuff.

♦ **Workmen's cafe/van**. These are way too greasy – everything in them is usually greasy. If you really have a hankering for a fry-up breakfast with all the trimmings, make sure you are only eating very, very small meals for the rest of the day and are going to do some sort of manual labour!

♦ **Wraps**. These are similar to crepes: it depends what is in them. Keep away from rich heavy fillings.

Let's see if Hope has been doing her homework on take-outs…

Hope arrived home to find her husband and daughter sitting at the kitchen table studying the menu for a new Indian restaurant that had just opened. There was not much anybody fancied in the fridge so they decided to give the Bombay Ball a call. Hope studied the menu quite carefully before ordering. She went with tandoori chicken, balti prawns, plain boiled pilau rice, a nan and curried vegetables for the three of them. She was careful to have only one plateful with mainly breast meat of the tandoori chicken, a spoonful of rice, a quarter of the nan and very little of the balti prawns and vegetable curry. She picked out the vegetables and prawns being careful to avoid the greasy sauces of these dishes. She drank a lot of water as well.

Her husband and daughter were impressed with her discipline. And even more impressed when she showed them how loose her jeans were. She was feeling good. And she was not depriving herself of what she liked to eat.

7

RESTAURANTS

Share a dessert.

The whole family, especially Hope, had been look-ing forward to their celebratory Sunday lunch at La Scala, the local Italian restaurant. The non-thinking Hope picked at the bread while she was deciding on her order of minestrone followed by her favourite pasta dish of penne cooked in a seafood cream sauce. To finish she had a rich strawberry cake with ice cream followed by cappuccino. She had a bit too much white wine and felt very sleepy by the time they left the restaurant. They had all planned on go-ing for a walk but instead opted for going home and putting their feet up!

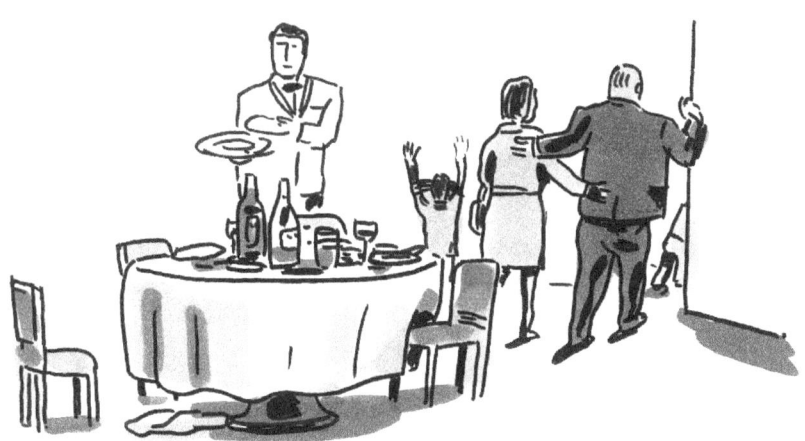

The Sunday lunch could have been just as enjoyable and healthy if Hope had made a few changes. Picking at the bread could have been fine if it was just a couple of bites. Minestrone is quite a heavy starter but can be alright if it is not eaten in vast quantities and is followed by something slightly lighter and not too rich. The pasta was OK and so was the seafood but the cream in the sauce was probably not the best idea, especially if it is going to be followed by more cream in the ice cream. If they had had slightly less wine tiredness might not have kicked in and their good idea of a walk would have happened.

Eating in restaurants should always be fun, enjoyable and sociable even when you are trying to lose weight or keep yourself in good shape. All the points I have mentioned in the previous chapters should still be applied. There is no reason to go into a restaurant and go berserk with your quantities!

Share a dessert.

However much you have or have not eaten during the meal there is never any reason for having a whole dessert to yourself. With the other courses it is harder to share, as your companions might not be too happy, but with dessert it is a different story. It is very acceptable these days to order one or two desserts with many more forks. Very few people insist on having a whole portion to themselves. Eating all of a sweet is the thing that can really leave you feeling full, and as you know it is much better to get up not feeling bloated. Cheese should also be included as a dessert and given the same treatment. Cheese is heavy and a lot of cheese is very heavy. If you are having tea or an infusion it is often worth checking if petits fours are served. These can often satisfy a craving for something sweet. If desserts are your favourite part of the meal, then disregard the above and eat very little of other courses and have your own dessert, but still try not to finish it!

Balance your meal.

This means that you should not have three heavy courses. If you choose a rich starter, try to have something lighter for a main course and 'share a dessert'. Remember that if you go for a light main course you should be aware of any vegetables that might come laced with butter or in a sauce. Green salad with oil and vinegar is a good side as is any steamed vegetable. But if you are just too tempted and overeat because it is so delicious just put it right the next day.

If in doubt, go for grilled fish, meat or vegetables.

Grilled food with no sauce is nearly always the best option, especially if you are trying to lose weight. Of course if you utterly loathe grilled food then ignore this. Most restaurants offer plain grilled food and if you do not always see something on the menu it is worth asking. Most meats or fish can be done in this way. Some foods are better than others; grilled salmon is far tastier than grilled cod and grilled lean steak is usually lighter than lamb chops unless all the fat is removed.

Restaurant tips

♦ Go easy on alcohol. I know I have already
mentioned this but it is very important especially when you are eating out and will
therefore probably have slightly more food
than usual. Be aware of your glass being
filled up and always make sure there is a
jug of water on the table so when you are
thirsty you do not reach for the wine/beer.

♦ If you like lager try the light variety and go
for it in moderation, but if you are able to
cut out beer and lager it would be better.
Especially if you have a lot of weight to lose.

♦ Get used to drinking diet versions of soft
drinks. They may taste strange at first but
once you are used to them you will never
want the regular kind (with at least 100
times the calories) again.

♦ Go easy on the bread and try to have it with
no butter. If you do want butter, remember
to spread it thinly. Again if you sit down
feeling ravenous and dive straight for the
bread, make sure that you remember you

have had some when ordering and eating.

♦ French food tends to have rich sauces – try to ask for them on the side or only eat some and try not to mop up the remains.

♦ Have two starters instead of a starter and main course. This is especially good to do at dinner as you should keep it light.

♦ Keep away from pasta with very creamy sauces – go for the tomato-based ones.

♦ Get a starter for the whole table and take a couple of bites. This is especially easy to do in Chinese, Indian, Mexican, Thai, Japanese and Greek restaurants.

♦ For salad dressing ask for oil, vinegar, salt and pepper to be brought to the table. Stay away from the blue cheese variety. If you hate oil and vinegar always get your chosen dressing on the side and go easy.

♦ When having Indian, Chinese or meals where you order collectively try to monitor how much you are eating. This collective ordering can be good if you eat sparingly:

you will get to taste a lot without eating a lot. But it can be harder to know how much you have eaten. Try to fill your plate up with a selection and once you have finished what is on it try to restrain yourself from filling it up again.

♦ Beware of buffet-style restaurants, especially the "all you can eat" variety – you always end up eating too much too quickly. If you are very disciplined they can be OK provided you select small amounts and do not go back for more.

♦ Salad bars in restaurants may seem a good option but some of the salads (especially potato and pasta) are really heavy, so go very easy. Anything green or raw is good.

♦ If you have time try to take as long in between courses as possible.

♦ If the cheese board looks amazing try very small bits of everything that looks good. Really have sample sizes.

♦ Ask how something is prepared if the menu does not clearly explain. If you want the particular piece of meat or fish and it is being prepared in a way that you do not want, you can always ask for it be made in a different way – plainly grilled – with the sauce served on the side.

♦ If you are having pizza or a meal that can be wrapped up, ask for a doggy bag. It is better to stop when you are full and leave the rest of it for another meal.

Ready to re visit *La Scala* with a wiser Hope...

*Hope was looking forward to going to La Scala
again. It was a fairly local restaurant and the day
was looking sunny so she suggested they all walk.
Her daughter needed a bit of heavy persuasion but
finally agreed, especially as it was her dad's birthday. He was very happy to go along with Hope's
walk. She seemed a different person these days. And
if more exercise was responsible – so be it. They all
really enjoyed the walk. Hope tried a tomato salad
to begin with and followed it with penne arrabiata.
She washed it down with a glass of champagne,
which took her the whole meal to finish. Cutting alcohol down and not out was OK.*

*She had decided to go all out for his birthday. And
at the end of the meal a column of waiters appeared
with one piece of her favourite strawberry cake with
a candle on top. Her husband and daughter devoured most of the cake but Hope managed to have
a couple of bites. Which actually was quite enough.*

8
TRAVEL

Do not throw caution to the wind.

They were all looking forward to their holiday by the sea in Italy. For the old Hope it would be sheer bliss to have a complete rest from cooking for everyone for two weeks. She was hoping to indulge herself with everything including her favourite pasta dishes, Italian ice creams and several bottles of Chianti.

There would be no running around for everyone, just plenty of very lazy time on a sunbed. She was planning on more sleeping by the sea than swimming in it. Any ideas of losing weight would have to wait! This was her time of the year to enjoy everything.

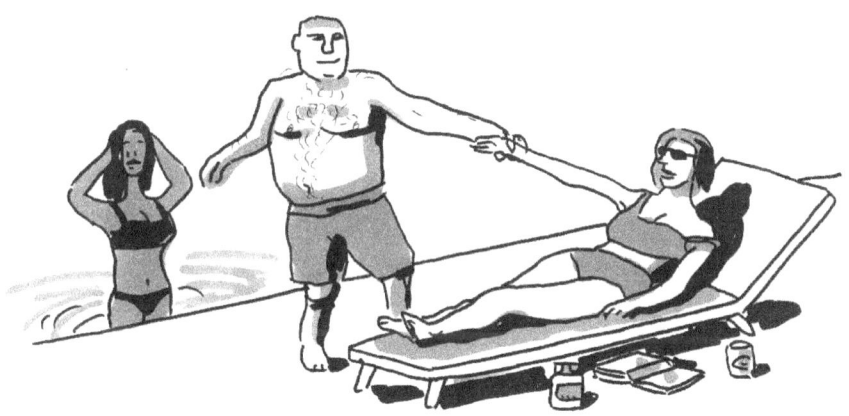

There is nothing wrong with Hope planning to enjoy everything – that is what holidays are for. What she had not thought of was that she could enjoy it all and not put on weight; in fact she could even lose weight if she remembered to carry on "eating less". Holidays should not be a time to put on weight.

There is no need to lose control of what you eat when you are away. The same basic rule still applies: eat less of whatever it is you are having. When travelling you should not be worried about trying new things – that is part of the fun. You can use the points mentioned already plus a few more. There is nothing more depressing than coming back from a trip either for work or pleasure and discovering that you have gained weight. You really can avoid that awful moment on the scales – if you want to enough!

Do not throw caution to the wind.

Do not suddenly think that because you are out of your normal environment that your newly acquired eating habits should be suspended. You can carry on with them and enjoy your trip.

Holidays can be a good time to lose weight.

This may sound surprising but it is true. While you are away you have more time to think about what you are eating. You should also be feeling less stressed, so if one of the reasons for overeating is stress, it is removed while you are away. Unless you are one of those people who find holidays highly stressful. In which case you will have to be extra careful. If you are staying in a hotel you will not have the temptation of a kitchen with a fridge. If you are renting a villa or apartment you will be starting with an empty larder. Do not feel tempted to fill it up unnecessarily.

Travel and seeing new places should be stimulating and your mind will hopefully be on your new surroundings and not your stomach.

Enjoy.

Food is an important part of travelling and part of the whole experience. As well as discovering new places it is good to discover new tastes. So there is no need to lessen the new experience – just the quantity! And if something is so delicious that you eat way too much, no matter. Just eat less the next day. That way you can "enjoy" everything.

Travel tips

♦ While you are actually travelling (in airports, stations, motorway services) the variety of food can be very limited, so you have to be careful. Airport food really varies. Some of the UK airports offer quite healthy stuff. US Airports are slowly improving but they do tend to be heavy on pizzas and hot dogs. Continental European, Asian and South American airports offer mainly local fare, often with a bit of international fast food thrown in. Try to share something with your fellow travellers if you have any. If not make your purchase last as long as possible.

♦ It really is not good to travel on a heavy stomach – eat lightly. It is particularly important to eat small amounts as you can get bored when travelling and end up eating more often just to pass the time.

♦ Drink as much water as possible – it not only fills you up but keeps you from dehydrating. Always buy water to take on a flight.

- ◆ Check if your plane/train provides food – if not make sure to take some food onboard. It is no good arriving somewhere starving as you will just eat too much when you reach your next meal.

- ◆ Airline meals: as a rule, never finish them. The desert should almost always never be eaten – one bite max!

- ◆ Citrus fruit is a healthy and good travel food. Try to travel with oranges – if you like them – especially on long-haul flights.

- ◆ Beware of hotel breakfasts, especially in countries like Italy and the USA where sugar products are very popular (sugary crois- sants, cakes, waffles, pancakes, French toast all with syrup and oodles of butter). If you like the above go very easy. Also be- ware of some egg dishes – they are often cooked in far too much fat.

- ◆ If you are curious to try something but not sure if it is really your thing and you are eat- ing with friends or family see whether any- one else is going for the dish and do a deal that you try their meal and they try yours.

- If you are on holiday in the sun and overeat a bit do a few more laps of the pool.

- When faced with mountains of the local un-healthy delicacy, just eat some of it and say you have a slightly delicate stomach. You can obviously use this excuse anywhere, anytime.

- If you can not understand the menu, look around at what other people are eating and find something that looks appetising and relatively healthy and point it out to your waiter.

- Limit the amount of fruit punches and cock-tails you have around the pool at happy hour.

- Skiing makes you hungry but try not to suc-cumb to too many hot chocolates with whipped cream.

- You have time to eat on holiday so make sure you eat slowly – long, leisurely meals are good.

- Try not to treat yourself to room service late

at night – even on holiday it is not good to eat late.

♦ If you are staying at a hotel that includes a set-meal supper/lunch you do not have to eat all the courses. Similarly at an all-inclusive resort you should restrain yourself and not go back to the buffet table for seconds and thirds!

♦ Remember, when eating out in America, that the portions are nearly always too large. But it is very acceptable to ask for anything to be boxed up and taken away – to be unwrapped when you are hungry and ready for a meal, otherwise you can end up snacking on the remains before the next meal. And one, two, three you have eaten the whole massive amount.

♦ In contrast to the American sizes are the French sizes, in fact most continental European sizes. Much better.

It's a whole year later and Hope and her family are off on holiday. Will she put into practice her new eating habits?

They are all going to a little fishing village near Jerez in southern Spain. For the first time they are renting a villa on the beach. It should suit everyone. Sandcastles for her toddler, local nightlife for her daughter and peace for Hope and her husband, with the odd visit to the local tapas bar. Hope has no desire to overindulge this year. She looks too good in her bikini. The first time she has worn one since having her daughter.

They really enjoy the visits to the local markets. She seems to have convinced everyone to eat healthily. They stock up on tomatoes, salad, vegetables, fruit, fish and local wine. Every meal is a delight. Tapas bars feel as if they were meant for Hope. All they serve is small portions. There is huge variety but not huge quantity. Spain is definitely the place for her.

When Hope gets home and goes on the scales she is elated. She has actually lost weight. On one of the best holidays of her life!

9

EXERCISE

Burn what you eat.

Our old Hope had forgotten to renew her membership to the gym and was feeling very guilty. She needed to carry on working out or there would be no exercise in her life. But her last few visits to the gym had been very hurried and she felt as if she was spending most of her time getting there, showering and getting home and her actual time working out was shrinking. She got a real high from physical exercise and she just wanted to do more and more. It was just a matter of finding the time!

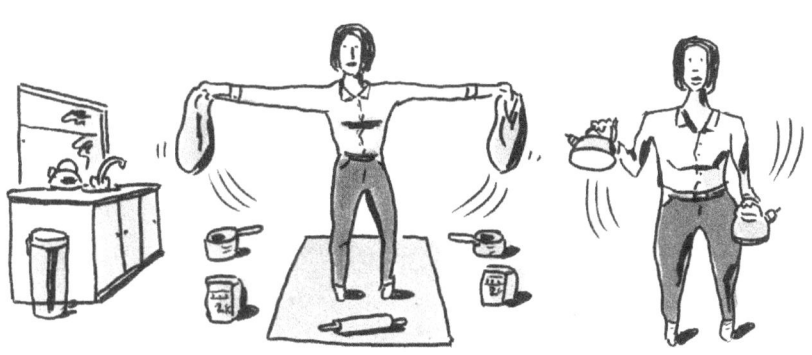

Hope scores high with her ambitious exercise plans, as long as they materialise into real activity. Time seems to be her enemy, so maybe she should be looking for a nearer gym or even finding some sort of work-out to do in her home.

I have never done any "formal" exercise – regular jogging or working out in the gym. This does not mean that it is wonderful not to. To those of you who do, carry on the good work. My exercise is just moving as much as I can, which is again based on nothing rigid or prescribed – just doing what you already do – but in this case more!

Burn what you eat.

This is really what exercise is all about – using up the calories that we take in. If you burn up more than you eat you will lose weight; if you burn up exactly what you take in you will stay the same weight and if you take in more than you use up you gain weight and get fat! All very obvious. It does not really matter what exercise you do as long as you do enough.

Exercise is in the little things as well as the big things.

What this means is that you can do a massive work-out in the gym for an hour or you can rush around the house or take several short walks. This is all exercise. Many people seem to be obsessed with the idea that there has to be a specific time to do structured exercise. The structured stuff is fine but not the only way to go. My way is all about exercise in the broadest sense – literally moving as much as you can.

Get up and go.

So much of what we do today is sedentary: sitting at a desk, watching TV, playing computer games, driving. We need to get into the habit of taking a break from our sitting position – just getting up and doing some small physical activity. Everything is designed to keep us in our chairs – remote controls, TV dinners, electronic door openers. You should try to "get up and go" somewhere, even if it is into another room or round the block, every hour, just to stretch your legs.

Exercise tips

♦ Walk instead of taking the car/bus/tube whenever you can, and if you see you have just missed a bus walk on to the next stop.

♦ If you live in a house, go up and down the stairs as much as possible.

♦ Do your own cleaning. This can be a good alternative to the gym. Doing a vigorous clean quite quickly becomes a work-out. It is very easy to break into a sweat. Especially if you give yourself a certain amount of time to clean. There are several advantages as well: you can chose when to do it, no travelling is involved, you save money and you can do as little or as much as you want.

♦ Always be the one to jump up and get something. The more you move the better. This does not mean that you should become everybody's servant. You get up when you want to, not when a lazy partner or child asks you!

♦ Take a long walk at the weekends or whenever you have the time. Try to have a regular time when you walk with a friend. Make it into a social thing, something you look forward to.

♦ If you have been sitting still for an hour, get up and move around. This is especially important if you are working at a desk.

♦ Do the ironing. Just another small activity that occupies you at home and so stops you eating and produces something.

♦ If you enjoy playing any sports, make sure that you give yourself time to do it. If you decide to take up a sport or activity again it is good to do it with someone else if you can: on days when you are not in the mood, another person can push you into action.

♦ Do not be deterred from doing exercise because you are feeling tired. Physical activity usually wakes you up and makes you feel good.

♦ If you are out for the evening, do more dancing than drinking.

- Gardening is really good exercise, especially mowing and digging.

- Whenever you can, sit upstairs on a double-decker bus – more stairs to go up and down!

- Whenever you can take the stairs instead of the lift.

- Walk up an escalator – do not just stand on one step.

- Treat moving walkways the same as escalators and keep walking.

- On summer holidays give yourself a target of how many laps you want to do each day in the pool and really do them!

- If you are having a break in a city get a good map and discover places on foot, not from a tour bus. In fact, try and walk whenever you can in a new city. It is a wonderful way of getting a feel for the place and working off the extra food you might eat while away.

- If you enjoy riding a bike – ride to work if you can.

- When taking the car somewhere don't mind parking some way away from your destination and walking.

- If you enjoy "formal" exercise carry on with it and incorporate some of these ideas into your life. The more you exercise the better.

- When speaking on the phone, use a cordless one and walk or pace round the room – that way the longer you talk the longer you walk.

Let's see if Hope is succeeding with her exercise plans…

Hope's life had really changed since she had bought herself a pedometer. She put it on each morning and constantly checked how many steps she was doing. To increase her walking she had moved her small home office to the top of the house. Suddenly she was going up and down the stairs loads of times every day. The more she did the climb the less she seemed to feel it.

She had taken to giving herself a time limit for hoovering the whole house. When she managed to stick to the deadline she felt as if she had done a long work-out at the gym. Suddenly she had a home gym that gave results.

Her other big change was doing the garden – well mainly mowing the lawn. She also enforced time limits on herself for this. At the end of the day if she had not clocked up enough steps she just walked up and down the stairs a few times. If that was not enough she dragged her partner out for a walk around the block. She had also continued with her membership to the local gym where she still worked out with friends. She was beginning to feel really good from all the extra-curricular exercise she was taking!

10

EVER AFTER

Never stop being aware of what you eat.

Hope had been at her goal weight for three weeks! She had been wearing the jeans she had worn before the children plus some new "thin" clothes. She had continued to be very careful with her portion sizes even during her celebratory dinner. She had been weighing herself daily for the first two weeks. During the third week she had indulged in a few too many glasses of wine. The daily weigh-in had been swapped for a weekly one. And she got a shock when she finally got on the scales. The alcohol had turned into extra pounds. She felt very fed up and FAT. In reality she had only put on two pounds (0.9 kilos). Would she be able to lose the pounds quickly and not add to them? She knew she could....

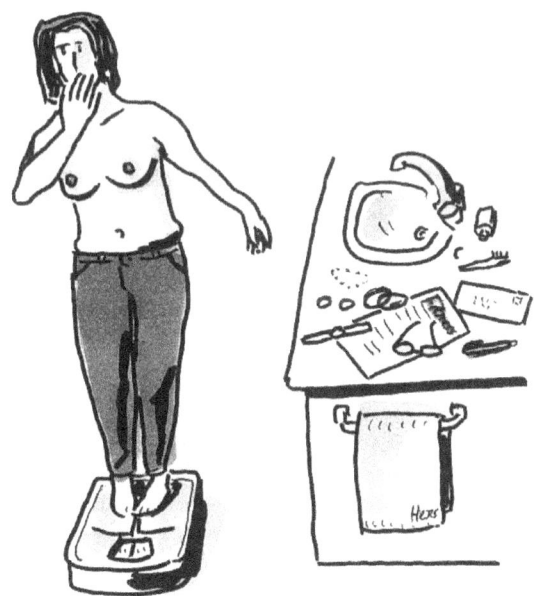

Hope had done well in getting down to her goal weight. She was definitely right to go out to treat herself to some new clothes and having a celebratory dinner was fine. What she has to be careful of is not letting the extra pounds stay on or, even worse, grow. So many people lose weight and then make the mistake of going back to their old eating habits and slowly it creeps back on.

A few simple rules can help here too.

Never stop being aware of what you eat.

If you carry on always being aware and following the rules in the previous chapters you should stay the way you want to be. By now, with luck, you should be thinking about food and exercise in the right way, so that it all just becomes part of how you live. The lifestyle change should have happened.

Enjoy feeling good.

You are at the weight you want to be, so feel good about it and enjoy the feeling. If you are about to eat something just for the sake of it, say no to yourself. Staying in shape is more important than having a piece of chocolate cake that you really do not have room for at the end of a big meal. Have one bite!

The "blue dot".

I was out to dinner with a friend and noticed he had an interesting blue dot on the face of his watch. I asked him about the dot. He said he got the dot from a stationery shop. I was puzzled. He explained he was someone who always watched what he ate. And by looking at the blue dot he was reminded about what to eat. A kind of "dot acupuncture". By the look of him, it seemed to be successful.

Weigh yourself every day.

Weighing yourself every day might be a little over the top for you – if so, fine – just hit the scales once a week or if your clothes feel the tiniest bit tight. If you are someone who will weigh yourself every day, then make sure you do it at the same time. If you are a woman do not weigh yourself during or just before or after your period. You can add pounds. By weighing yourself daily or weekly you will notice the smallest weight gain and can deal with it quickly before it gets out of control. Remember, the scales do not lie!

Ever-after tips

♦ Treat yourself to some new clothes.

♦ Give your "big" clothes to charity, or if that is too scary put them in the loft or in a box.

♦ Carry on eating the way you have been eating, but allow yourself a little bit more.

♦ Carry on exercising in the same way.

♦ Do not suddenly increase your alcohol intake.

♦ Always have "diet" drinks.

♦ Always have semi-skimmed milk.

♦ Look after your body (body cream, home facials, etc).

♦ Learn to listen to your body and eat when you are hungry.

♦ If you put on a little weight (do not panic) just lose it!

- If you are a routine kind of person then maybe eating the same things each day would work for you. I have certain things that I have on a daily basis and this works well. It is said we are creatures of habit so maybe give it try. If this sounds boring, ignore it.

- If you feel tired or below par then check that you are eating enough of the right things.

- Since you want to stay as you are, that means not losing weight as well as not putting it on. So make sure that if you are having a very energetic time you eat enough.

The big question. Has Hope managed to get back to and stay at her goal weight?

Hope is eating three meals a day and even snacking. And, after losing the two pounds she has been the same weight for three months. She weighed herself every day. She even had the confidence finally to chuck out all her fat clothes. As usual she had gone to her parents for Christmas lunch and Boxing Day supper. Not an ounce of weight had been gained. It had been a beautiful, crisp Christmas and she had encouraged everyone to go for a very long walk. Her husband had given her a new watch and the first thing she did was stick a pink spot on the dial!

11

THE AGONY

Frequently unasked questions.

Hope impressed everyone she met with her weight loss. Suddenly she was becoming a kind of diet guru for all her overweight friends. She began to realise just how interested everyone was to find out about her "miracle diet" and once she started talking the conversations just went on and on. She had hardly ever spoken to anyone about wanting to lose weight and now she so regretted it. Once her secret was out everyone wanted to share it with her. They seemed to be asking her the most obvious questions and she was more than happy to answer all of them. She had become a kind of eating agony aunt. It all helped her to stay on track with her reformed eating habits. If only she had talked about it before – but at least better late than never!

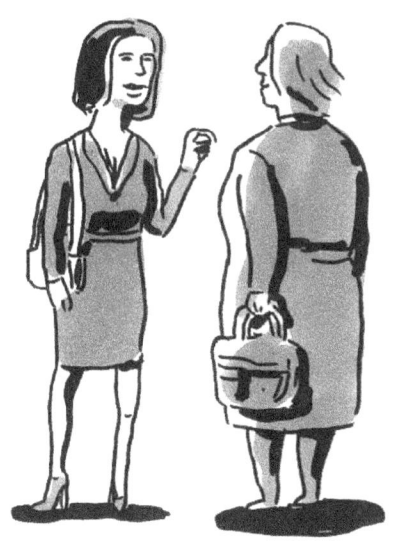

What Hope experienced just shows how often people are inhibited to ask even the most obvious questions.

Here are some questions that I was asked…

Is going on a diet a waste of time?

Going on a "diet" is not a waste of time if you lose weight instead of gaining it. I have two very different friends who went on diets at roughly the same time.

One strictly followed a well-known diet. I saw her, after a gap of several months, and remarked that she had lost loads of weight and looked great. I saw her again a few months later and she said she had put a lot back on and would not go on the diet again: as she really had not felt healthy at all, and more to the point in the long term she had hardly changed her weight. She weighed 144 pounds (65 kilos) before starting the diet: 133 pounds as soon as she came off it; and within a short period she was back to 142 pounds. The sums are easy. She had lost just 2 pounds after all the sacrifices.

Another friend managed to lose 21 pounds by simply creating her own eating plan from a selection of diets. That worked for her. She lost her weight and is keeping it off. Her only remark to me was that she did not want to get too thin. She has really cracked it.

So, the answer is to find a way of eating that works for you. So many people are looking for a miracle diet that will solve all their weight problems. I remember countless strange diets that my mother went on. They ranged from eating a grapefruit before each meal of hyper quantities of protein to having double cream instead of single. It's obvious that that kind of crazy eating might possibly help you lose a bit of weight, but (trust me) it goes back on really, really fast. Still in search of the perfect way to lose weight mum went to health farms where she was reduced to eating greenery and more greenery. But she never lost the pounds, even after a week sequestered in these fat farms. Why? She sneaked out to the teashop in the local village for toasted current buns and butter! As you can see most of the extreme diets really are a waste of time – even if you are staying in a health farm you have to believe you could possibly live the rest of your life on what you are eating.

However, going on the right diet for you is absolutely not a waste of time. Try all the things in the previous chapters and see what happens. Think of your diet as an adventure, not a chore.

Isn't it all about metabolic rate anyway?

No it isn't 99.9% of the time, unless you have some clinical problems. People who say that are often trying to kid themselves that some are just born lucky and that they were born unlucky. Wrong: some were born active and not partial to overeating and others were born a bit lazy and partial to overeating. There were far fewer fat people let alone morbidly obese people during the war when there was rationing and less sedentary pastimes. The only thing that has changed is how much and what people eat, not the way their bodies process the stuff.

It is no coincidence that Americans are the fattest nation and an alarming proportion of American children are overweight. Theirs is the land with the biggest portions and the biggest people. Their metabolic rates are no different to the French or English. It doesn't take rocket science – or even a docufilm like "Supersize Me", in which a person systematically eats supersized portions – to know that if you eat mega-amounts you will get mega-shaped.

An interesting thing happened when researchers observed several people that they put on an eating re-gime of unhealthy food for a month and forbade them to do any exercise. These people spent their time watching television and being inactive. At the end of the month most of the group had put on a sig-nificant amount of weight; but a couple of them had gained very little. The reason for this became clear when tapes of their actions over the month were played back. The ones who had gained little weight had walked constantly as they spoke on the phone, tapped their feet on the ground while watching tele-vision and constantly shifted around in their seats.

Systematic research on this "fidget factor" has been done at the Mayo Clinic in Rochester, Minnesota. There scientists have taken underwear to a new level, designing it to measure every tiny movement. Sensors embedded in racy-looking cutouts at the crotch and backside and special pockets capture the slightest activity. Literally millions of measure-ments later, the scientists can establish just how much energy is used in the most inconspicuous ways. Even chewing gum burns up 11 calories an hour if you chew six pieces at a time! Bottom line; the restless and fidgety can use up 350 calories a day more than their inactive – and fatter – fellow guinea pigs in the Mayo designer underwear. Over time this daily difference is enough for fat people to take off 30 to 40 pounds (14 to 18 kilos) a year. Since becoming aware of the "fidget factor" I have surreptitiously been observing friends. The nervous fidgeters are definitely the leanest. There are a few unlucky people who are born with medical problems. But these are the unfortunate few, compared with the millions who just eat too much.

I keep my own weight down but my partner has trouble doing the same. What should I do?

This problem is all too familiar. I keep my weight down and my partner does not.

You should probably do what I fail to do: stop mentioning eating less, stop trying to impose my will and stop nagging. The secret seems to be to remind them gently to eat less without making them feel like a deprived child. My partner suggests that it is good to discuss it in a civilised way well away from the food area. Talk about foods that can be eaten quite liberally and others that should be moderated. Invent a word that can be used instead of "eat less".

Eating is enjoyable, and the fun must not be taken out of it. If you are serving their food, try to fill the plate with healthy food and leave only a little space for the not-so-healthy stuff. They should feel they have a reasonable plateful and not feel deprived. Explain that there are no good or bad foods, just foods you should eat more or less of.

A good time to try to help is on holiday. You will see exactly what they eat and how much of it. When everyone is relaxed is a good time to look at life generally, including getting fit and changing eating habits. Just remember not to be too dogmatic and let your partner do a lot of the talking. I'm sure they already know what you have to say on the subject!

Remember you are controlled enough to keep your weight down and they are not. Suggest goals with them that are reachable and suit them – not you. Ultimately your partner has to want to keep the weight off for themselves. Whatever you say will have no effect unless they want it to.

Good luck.

I know what I am supposed to eat (less!) but I cannot manage the discipline. What do you recommend?

For a start do not think of managing discipline. Just think about saying no to your urge to overeat. The more you say no the easier it will get. I promise.

Here are a few reminders on how to deal with all that scrumptious temptation.

As soon as you feel full, remove your plate and wash it up. Once the food is gone you will have removed temptation. Make sure you put the leftovers in the bin or down the waste disposal at once. If you want to keep them, cover them tightly with cling film and put them to the back of the fridge.

Walk out of the kitchen if you think you will start picking at food because you are bored. Boredom is your enemy. Give yourself little time to be bored and you will eat less.

Only eat in the kitchen. Not in the TV room, the study or even the bedroom. The fewer places where food is available the less temptation is in your path.

Before you pop something into your mouth – think. Would I rather be slim or eat this? I bet the answer is slim. So do not put it in your mouth but instead walk away and congratulate yourself on saying "no".

It is really hard when you are seated with a wonderful meal in front of you and you know you should eat less. Start by deciding that you will not have seconds. You can congratulate yourself on sticking to that. If you feel in a particularly positive mood you could decide to leave some food on the plate when you think you have eaten enough. Do not feel bad if you do neither because it is all just so delicious. Just eat less later or the next day. Some days it will be easier to manage discipline. Make the most of them.

The discipline is the hardest thing to crack. But if you really want to say no and stick to it, you will. It is not like smoking, where no means none. No just means less. Remember that "no just means less". The discipline is only over size.

I can stick to the sensible eating for a while, but then it all goes wrong. How do I make it permanent?

First of all stop thinking about it as sensible. Sensible is boring and unsexy. Think about eating "your way" or even "your crazy way". That sounds more fun, less rigid and totally personal.

Eat your way most of the time and if sometimes you go wrong and eat too much – no matter. Just eat less the next day. If it goes wrong the next day just eat less the next. Do not feel that simply because you have deviated it is the end of your weight loss or the beginning of vast weight gain. Just weigh yourself and put the damage in perspective.

The longer you maintain your new eating habits the easier it will be. You will soon know what you can eat, instinctively, before you gain weight.

Remember, it is all about eating what you want, but less.

I don't do my own shopping. My partner buys the wrong things. What would you advise?

Why don't you suggest that you go with her? If she normally goes when you are unable to, suggest that you find a time when you can once go together. That must be possible, unless you live in the middle of nowhere. Plenty of supermarkets are open 24 hours. I am not suggesting that you plan a 2am visit to the aisles!

On this visit try to steer her into buying food that you want. You may find she puts up a bit of a fight. Old food shopping habits can be hard to change. It is up to you to make her realise just how important it is to you.

If a joint shopping trip is out of the question, you need to sit her down and explain that you want to eat in a more healthy way. Before you have your talk make a list of what you want her to buy. Make sure that she takes your list on her next shopping trip.

If she still ends up buying the wrong things you could take the matter into your own hands and ask that she gives you the money she would have spent on your food. Then you are totally responsible for buying your own food. Remember that if you are buying for yourself you do not need to buy family-sized packs of anything.

A word of warning. Make sure that whatever she buys with you, or whatever you buy, gets eaten. Trust me, she will be pretty fed up if you fill the fridge with your food and then chuck out much of it when the sell-by dates run out.

I am sure that if your partner is a reasonable kind of person and realises that you just want to eat in a better way, she will comply. You might even end up educating her on the right things to buy.

You say breakfast is the most important meal of the day but I can't manage to eat it. Does it matter?

I wonder why you cannot manage to eat it. Is it because you do not have time, you are not hungry early in the morning or do you think that by missing it you will stay thin?

If you really don't have time – make time. If you are really not hungry then have a mid-morning breakfast. If you think missing it will keep you slim or make you lose weight – wrong.

But if you can manage to miss breakfast, eat well for the rest of the day and not gain weight over a long period of time, missing it does not matter.

The important thing is to eat in a way that satisfies you and keeps you slim. And if missing breakfast works for you then stay with it. But I maintain that if you eat a light supper you will be craving for breakfast!

If, however, you do not feel satisfied and your weight yo-yos – it matters. And maybe the time has come to get up earlier and make a huge effort to eat breakfast or have a mid-morning breakfast. I always think routine is helpful, so decide on a "breakfast plan of action" and try to stick to it.

Many people I talk to have very little breakfast on weekdays but often have the works at the weekend because they have time. It seems, so often, to come down to time. It's obvious, but the only way to make time for breakfast is to get up earlier.

I buy sensible food but my children complain and say there is nothing good to eat. What do I do?

Nothing. It might sound tough but do not give in to them.

My children complain all the time that there are no good snacks in the house. By good snacks they mean crisps (I buy one multi-pack of 10 small packets and that has to last my two children plus their friends all week), pop tarts, biscuits, chocolate bars, strange coloured cereal and all other foods of this ilk.

When they complain just list all the things there are to eat. Fruit is one of the best snacks and if you buy loads of fruit and leave it in a prominent place they will eat it if they are really hungry. Toast is a good snack, in moderation, and there are many toppings both sweet and savoury. Cereals of the non-colourful variety with semi-skimmed milk are OK. Small pots of yogurts are popular.

Tell them you only buy good food.

Children should not start their adult life being fat – it is a disadvantage and it is a parent's job to help them eat well! Explain all this to them. If they are older they should understand and if they are small they should just eat what you buy.

Most children will get their share of junk food when they are out or with friends. You really do not have to import it into the house. Children tend to complain less about wanting junk or ready meals for main meals unless they have been brought up on a diet of chicken fingers and ready-made chips.

One day your children will thank you for the sensible food you buy.

Should I pay attention to things I read in glossy magazines about eating?

No. Except when you see something that endorses how you are eating – the blindingly obvious way! Glossies tend to deal with eating either by writing long, slightly preachy pieces that are nutritionally based. So if you like these, read them. But do not change your eating plan if it is working. Or they publish diets under titles like "Lose 500 pounds in 34 days" or "Eat dried figs and cabbage on alternate days for the body you want" or "The underwear diet" or even "The revolutionary new imagine yourself thin diet". If you want to be amused, glance at these with the proviso that you will not in any circumstances be tempted. Magazines are meant to be sold and any eye-catching diet is of great interest.

The only time I ever pay attention to stuff in glossy magazines is when they interview real people who have lost a tremendous amount of weight and then kept it off. These articles are proof that it can be done. These people have almost always changed their whole approach to eating and exercising. If you want to be inspired or encouraged, these are the articles to zoom in on. Not the fad or extreme diet ones. Also, beware of articles that share with you what the stars eat and how they keep their perfect bodies. Most conveniently omit to tell you how many times they have been under the surgeon's knife.

So, don't pay attention but have fun looking.

How do I know when I am the right weight? You say "eat more" but how much more?

You could look at a chart that gives height with a range of good body weights next to it. But I think you know that you have reached your right weight when you feel happy with your body and you look good in all your clothes. Friends and family will usually be pretty honest and tell you if you are looking great or gaunt.

People decide on their right weight in a variety of ways. Many go back to a time when they felt they were their perfect size, usually when they were way younger. Others have actually kept a piece of clothing that they are determined to get into again. Most people know deep down what they should weigh. Knowing what the scales should say is not the problem. Getting to what they say can be.

Some people have maybe three sections in their wardrobes that hold "thin clothes", "fat clothes" and "most of the time clothes". If you really change your eating you should be able to have the confidence to get rid of all the sections except "thin clothes". A wardrobe of only "thin clothes" really means you have done it!

OK, so you have reached your perfect size and you want to increase your food intake without getting bigger. This is the most important time: the transition between "eating to lose and eating to stay". You can try being slightly less disciplined with yourself. For example, if you want seconds, have them. Eat slightly more heavy foods if you want to. Splurge occasionally when you go out for a wonderful meal. Weigh yourself regularly, though. You will soon have a feel for how much you should eat.

The more exercise you do the more you should eat. It's that obvious thing again – eat more than you use and you will gain, eat what you use and you will stay the same!

Isn't it wrong to have me worry so much about my weight? Shouldn't I just be happy as I am?

It depends just how fat you really are. If you are 7 to 14 pounds (3 to 6 kilos)) overweight and honestly feel happy about it, then fine. Be happy and do not worry. If you are hugely overweight then I do not believe that you can really be happy about it; plus it is bad for you.

You so often hear people say "I should be liked and

respected for who I am inside, not just how I look".
Maybe, in an ideal world. But the brutal truth is that
most people make snap decisions about others and
looks cannot help coming into it. Our society is becoming even more obsessed with looks. I am not
saying this is good or bad, just stating the facts. Big
is really not beautiful!

Being very overweight can hamper you in getting
jobs, finding a partner, lowering your self esteem,
and in the extreme threaten your health.

I have yet to meet an honest overweight person who
is happy and does not really want to lose weight. A
TV programme "Fatland", filmed about half a dozen
Brits going on holiday to an idyllic beach resort in
Mexico for obese people. The beds were reinforced,
the hammocks were reinforced, the beach chairs
were reinforced and the showers were made extra
large. Yet even in these perfect surroundings it took
a lot of coaxing to get some of the holidaymakers to
expose themselves in swimwear. None of these
overweight people seemed at all happy with their
size despite being subjected to an overweight
American who made her living telling tubbies to be
positive about being fat.

Just look at the hundreds of articles that show be-
fore-and-after pictures of the fatty transformed into

the slim swan. These transformations happened only because they were unhappy as they were and decided to do something about it.

Of course in an ideal world you should be happy just as you are. But in the real world you're more likely to like the way you are if you're not fat!

*One of Hope's friends, who worked on a local pa-
per, was so impressed with her impromptu agony-
aunt skills that she asked her if she would like to do
it professionally. This was a fantastic offer given at
just the right time. Hope had been feeling for a
while that her old job was going nowhere. Her
friend arranged a meeting with the editor and bingo
she was the new eating agony aunt for the "Voice".
She was now know as "Body Babe".*

12

THE ECSTASY

Blindingly obvious benefits.

Hope had never been so happy before. She felt like a teenager again. She could share clothes with her daughter, not that her teenager saw this as particularly good. Her marriage was thriving. Her husband looked at her very differently these days. And she felt so good about herself. She almost found it impossible to believe that just by losing those extra pounds she had been reborn. She had energy to do long walks, go up and down the stairs without feeling as if she would collapse and even go jogging with her husband, whom she had convinced to eat less.

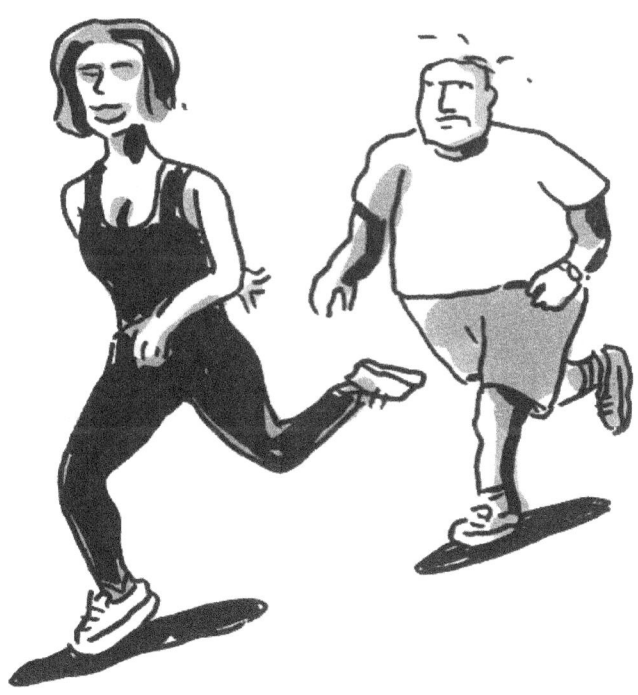

Amazing to think that all Hope needed to do to feel so good was to follow a few simple rules. She felt like a new person, and so can you. If you remember nothing else from this book, keep in mind the main message from each chapter.

When you are shopping remember that what you buy is what you eat.

Of all the shopping tips if, you are mindful of this, you will be on your way.

Remember to have breakfast.

This is the most important thing about breakfast – to have it!

It is important not to miss lunch.

It is easy to miss lunch or have it late as a kind of "sunch" (supper & lunch). Please don't.

Supper is the meal to eat the least of.

Think simple, small supper.

Think before you snack.

Be aware of all the reasons why you want to snack. The only one that justifies snacking is, believe it or not, hunger – real, tummy-rumbling hunger!

When you have a take-out, do the ordering yourself.

This is when it is advisable to have control over what arrives on the doorstep: a kind of home-delivery version of "what you order is what you eat".

Share a dessert in a restaurant.

Desserts seem to be getting bigger, so this should be easy – and more vital.

When you travel do not throw caution to the wind.

You really can eat well on holiday without going berserk. It is satisfying to get home and onto the scales and not have a horrible shock.

Burn what you eat.

If you eat a lot, exercise a lot.

Never stop being aware of what you eat.

Just keep a check on what you eat.

Imagine that, like Hope, you have absorbed these rules and have been living by them for a while. What will be different about your life? Plenty…

Looking good.

You will feel great. It's amazing how good you can feel inside when you are happy with the way you look on the outside.

Think about all those reality makeover shows – they have one thing in common. The victim always feels more confident and ready to take on the world after they have been made over and look good. You will feel good without enduring the scrutiny of the nation's telly-watchers.

Obviously, not being overweight is not the only thing that increases people's confidence. But for better or worse, we live in a society that is becoming more and more "lookist". Research quoted in the *International Herald Tribune* shows that obese woman get 17% lower wages than women of average weight and that dishy professors get better evaluations from their students.

Let's face it, looking good was one of the main aims of getting into shape, and you are there!

Feeling healthy.

Feeling healthy and fit will have the biggest impact on your life. You will have more energy for doing things. Walking will no longer feel like a chore. Going up and down the stairs will not puff you out. You will feel younger and, with luck, live longer.

America, which sadly has a huge obesity problem, also has extreme examples of fatties who have managed to lose weight. An edition of *People* magazine featured several spectacular slimmers. One woman lost 75 pounds (34 kilos) and from being a confirmed couch potato she is now a weekend wilderness guide. Another lost 240 pounds and says the best part is "feeling good about myself and doing things I thought I'd never be able to do". And one man, who lost 80 pounds, found that his life had changed dramatically. "One thing I thought I'd never do in a million years," he explained, "my wife and I opened our (Christmas) presents and went out jogging for an hour... I am so thankful I did this."

Don't worry. Few people can be such super-slimmers. But they show the art of the possible – and how much healthier people can feel. Feeling healthy inspires people to be more active and keeping active keeps you fit and lean. A healthy circle.

Being in control.

Congratulations! You are in control.

Unless you are having a slightly out-of-control day – and we all have those. You now decide when to eat, what to eat and how much to eat. If you want to have a blowout meal you know you can because you can just eat less the next meal or day. Food is not scary now. Eating does not mean getting fat; it just means doing something you need to do. Food is something you can really enjoy. You know that if you want to pick at something it is probably because you are bored so you just find something to do instead. You have learnt to control your comfort-eating pangs.

And you know that if you go out of control sometimes, as we all do, it doesn't matter. You will soon be in control again.

Clothes shopping.

For many people this is probably a very superficial benefit. But for the vainer amongst us, unfortunately, it is a real plus. Shopping is now fun. for those of us who enjoy it! If you don't – skip this bit of ecstasy. For those of you who get pleasure from this frivolous activity – read on…

Now you actually enjoy picking out clothes – you look good in them. The dreaded changing rooms are not such a nightmare. The mirrors are not an unpleasant reminder of what you look like but a confirmation of how good you are looking. Sadly, there are always a few mirrors that manage to make you look slightly deformed or too tall and thin. Beware of these.

You also have the perfect excuse to treat yourself to a new wardrobe. Nothing fits!

Food for enjoyment.

You are at your ideal weight so enjoy your food. We have to eat to live, so it is a real plus to be able to get pleasure from it and remain the same size.

You know what to eat and how much to eat to keep to the weight you want to be, so have fun with food. You are how you want to be so you really can experiment more with new flavours and tastes. Because maybe now you naturally eat small amounts and enjoy them.

If you are invited to someone for a meal – enjoy. If you are taken to a good restaurant – enjoy. Each meal should be enjoyed.

Discovering new places.

You probably think this is a weird by-product of losing weight, but it is a really good one. The more you walk, even locally, the more new places you discover. But that is nothing compared to when you travel further. As soon as you know you are going to visit a new city, get a map. Walking somewhere you don't know really gives you a feel for it.

The more you walk the more you will want to walk. Plus, the more you walk in a foreign place, the more foreign food you can treat yourself to!

Live longer.

This is not a sure-fire way of prolonging life. But it can help. Scientists are even predicting that if the obesity trends carry on children will be dying before their parents. So help your children to eat like you do. That way you have a chance of them looking out for you in your old age.

Work done at the University of California at Berkeley suggests that we might be able to live longer by only a 5% reduction in calories, but sadly the study was done on mice! More studies showed that possibly it would work on other animals and humans if we fasted every other day! Forgetting the mice study, if you eat less, exercise and keep your weight down you should, with luck, live a bit longer.

Forget fads and yo-yos.

By now all those crazy diets are in the bin and you know the right way to eat. No more pumpkin seed diets. In fact, the very words used by this slimmer of the year 2005 were "How I lost eight stone (112 pounds) in 18 months....by dropping the fad diets". No more yo-yo diets. *The Times* (of London) reported that trials of a vaccine against obesity were about to start in Switzerland. The vaccine consists of an antibody against ghrelin, a small protein that regulates appetite. Interestingly, ghrelin has also been implicated in yo-yo dieting. Overweight people who lose weight develop higher levels of ghrelin which encourages them to eat more and put the weight back on again. And, for those who can't wait for the vaccine there are even more extreme ways to reduce the levels of ghrelin. By having operations to reduce their stomach size. Apparently ghrelin levels are reduced as a result of the operation.

Feel proud of yourself. You got to this point without trial vaccines and surgery!

So, by now you should know never to be tempted by a fad diet.

So now you know.

Eureka! You know what to do to control your body. So obvious, you really knew it all along.

Eat less and exercise more. It's as simple as that. Meanwhile, the ultimate compliment was given to Hope…

Out of the blue, Hope received a phone call from a publisher who had been taken with the "Body Babe" column. He asked Hope if she would be interested in writing a book about her weight loss and how she was keeping it off. He believed it would help a lot of people.

Acknowledgements

Thank you to Daniel for believing I could write this and then being the best editor. To Clio for transforming my erratic layout into a book. To Josh for living with less food than he would have liked. To Andrew Franklin and David Grossman for their support. And a huge thank you to Jim Sillavan for his wonderful artwork.

Gaby Franklin is a businesswoman and interior designer. She lives in London with her slightly overweight husband and two children.

www.thedietillusion.com

www.ingramcontent.com/pod-product-compliance
Lightning Source LLC
Chambersburg PA
CBHW060625290526
45793CB00001B/149